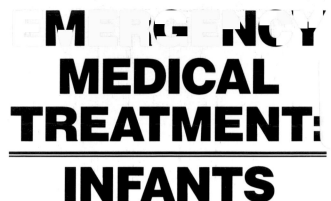

EMERGENCY MEDICAL TREATMENT: INFANTS

A HANDBOOK OF WHAT TO DO IN AN EMERGENCY TO KEEP AN INFANT ALIVE UNTIL HELP ARRIVES

By Stephen N. Vogel, M.D. and David H. Manhoff

PUBLISHER'S NOTE: This book is not intended to take the place of qualified help in the event of an emergency. In any emergency, call for qualified help immediately. This book is meant to provide you with life saving procedures until that qualified help arrives. It is also recommended that you take a certified CPR and first aid course.

TRANSMISSION OF HIV/AIDS AND HEPATITIS B VIRUS: The rescuer who responds in an emergency should be guided by the moral and ethical values of preserving life. In responding to an emergency, do what you think is best. The American Heart Association notes that if you are in doubt about exposure and won't initiate mouth-to-mouth ventilation, call for ambulance, open the airway, skip rescue breathing (mouth-to-mouth) and do chest compressions. If possible, prepare yourself by having personal protective equipment available (gloves & mouth barrier with one-way valve).

> The procedures as described in this book are based upon and follow the American Heart Association guidelines for Basic Life Support.

OTHER BOOKS AVAILABLE:
EMERGENCY MEDICAL TREATMENT: INFANTS / CHILDREN / ADULTS
EMERGENCY MEDICAL TREATMENT: ADULTS
EMERGENCY MEDICAL TREATMENT: CHILDREN
TRATAMIENTO MEDICO DE EMERGENCIA PARA NINOS
TRATAMIENTO MEDICO DE EMERGENCIA PARA INFANTES
TRATAMIENTO MEDICO DE EMERGENCIA PARA ADULTOS
MOSBY'S OUTDOOR EMERGENCY MEDICAL GUIDE

ISBN: 0-916363-01-5 Revised 1993
Technically reviewed by the National Safety Council.

While the information and recommendations contained in this publication have been compiled from sources believed to be reliable, the author, publisher and the National Safety Council make no guarantee as to, and assumes no responsibility for, the correctness, sufficiency, or completeness of such information and recommendations. Other or additional measures may be required under particular circumstances.

A Mosby Lifeline imprint of Mosby-Year Book, Inc.

Published by
Mosby-Year Book, Inc.
11830 Westline Industrial Drive
St Louis, MO 63146

Prevention

Automobile Safety

Infants weighing up to 20 lbs. should be in an infant safety seat which is designed to face towards the rear. Follow the manufacturer's instructions carefully. If car seats are used incorrectly, they will not protect the child. Read automobile owner's manual for any special instructions. Infants should ride in the back seat of the car, in the middle, if possible.

Fire Safety

Smoke detectors should be used on each level of your home, located at the top of each set of stairs and between the bedrooms. Test detectors once a month. Every home should have at least two working fire extinguishers. Keep in the kitchen and in the master bedroom.

Flame Resistant Sleepwear — Read the label on the wash product you use carefully. Soap washes out the flame retardant in material. You should wash in warm water with phosphate detergent. Do not use bleach or fabric softeners. Do not iron. Borax is a flame retardant and may be used in your laundry to restore protection.

Burns

Hot Liquids — Never carry a child and a hot liquid (coffee, tea) at the same time. Don't allow children near you in the kitchen while you are cooking. Always use the back burners on the stove, and turn any handles to the side, out of child's reach. Set water heater temperature at 110 degrees.

Hot Surfaces — When wall or floor heaters are in use, place child in a crib, playpen, or highchair.

Other burn prevention — use outlet covers for all electric outlets not in use; unplug appliances when not in use (don't allow appliance cords to dangle); use cold water vaporizers; keep all hazardous substances in a locked storage area, do not allow child to chew on electric cords.

Falls

Even a newborn infant can wiggle, squirm and push with their feet. Never leave them on a changing table, bed or other high place unless you have one hand on them at all times. When the child is older, they can climb up to high places, but they can't climb down.

Stairs — Keep stairs clear of toys, shoes, and other clutter. Check that carpeting is tacked down. If child is under three years old, use gates at the top and bottom of all stairways. Do not use accordion type gate, as a child may catch their fingers in it. Check that bannister posts are no more than 6″ apart, so child doesn't fall through.

Cribs — Don't leave the bumper pad or stuffed animals in the crib once child can stand. Leave the side rails up and the mattress in the lowest position when the child is in the crib. There should be no more than 2⅜″ between slats, and no more than two finger widths between the mattress and side of the crib (stuff the space if there is no more room). Remove any corner post extensions if they are higher than the side of the crib, and remove all hanging toys once the child can pull himself up. Once the child has climbed out or fallen over the rail, it is time to take the crib down.

Shopping Carts — Place child only in the seat provided in the shoppig cart. Secure them with strap and buckle. Never leave child alone in cart, as they may try to climb out or cart may tip over.

Choking

Food — Should be cut in very tiny pieces. A child's throat is the size of *their* little finger. Children under four should not be given peanut butter (it may "glue" the throat closed) or raisins. They should also not be given hot dogs, grapes, peanuts, popcorn or carrots.

Never prop a bottle while feeding an infant, as liquid will continue to flow out, even if the infant stops swallowing. Keep child seated while eating. Do not give small child food while riding in the car. If they were to choke, you may not realize it in time.

Small Objects — Small toy parts, coins, buttons, pen caps, safety pins, marbles, rings and earrings are often placed in the mouth. Keep away from child. Small round batteries are especially dangerous if swallowed. Keep purses, which contain these items, out of sight and out of reach.

Toys (size) — Check all toys for size of parts. Many toys have small parts that infants can choke on. If a toy or part can fit through a toilet paper tube, it is too small.

Balloons — *Uninflated or parts of burst balloons are the number one non-food item children choke on and die from.* Children may bite or burst an inflated balloon. Part of it may go down in the child's trachea, causing them to choke. Obstructed airway maneuvers do not work for balloons.

Water Safety

Bath — *Never leave infant alone in a bath tub for even a few seconds.* Children can drown in just a few inches of water very quickly.

Toilet/Buckets — Keep toilet lid down and clamped. Children enjoy water play, and may lean over too far and fall in. They are top heavy and cannot get out. Likewise, never leave a filled bucket.

Lake/Pool — Always designate *one person* to watch your child (if you cannot). More children drown when they are being watched by more than one person (each think the other is watching). Most children who drown, do so in residential pools — usually their own. Most fall in by riding a toy into the pool, or while playing too close to the edge. Do not use water wings as a safety device. Empty small wading pools after use.

General Household Safety

Playpens — Always have the sides up, so the child can't become enmeshed. Check that all hinges are secure so child's finger can't get caught.

Pillows, Blankets, Comforters, Bedspreads, Waterbeds — An infant can suffocate on a pillow. Just as with a waterbed, the sides may cover the nose and mouth. Infants can easily become entangled in bedspreads and comforters, and strangle themselves or suffocate.

Plastics bags — Tie bag in knots and throw away after use.

Older Children's Toys, Food, Etc. — Keep older children's toys and food away from infants and small children, as these items may be dangerous. Children should not run, walk or play while eating, or if they have a toy, toothbrush or lollipop in their mouth.

Unattended infant (phone call, doorbell, other children) — Never leave an infant unattended for any reason, at any time, unless they are in a crib or playpen.

Kitchen — Drawers and cupboards should have safety locks. Never leave sharp knives or appliance blades on the counter. Do not place highchair near a counter (child can push off) or a stove.

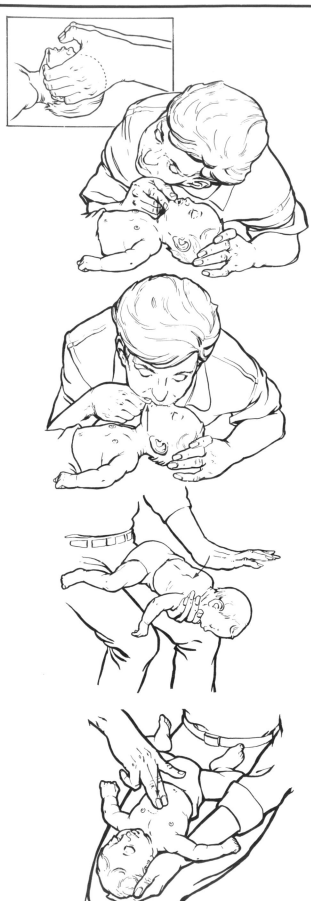

Gently tap or shake infant. If infant does not respond, shout for help.

1 Open airway, check breathing.

Lay infant on back. If you must roll infant on back, keep (support) head and neck in straight line. Tilt head back gently (not too far), lift chin slightly. Make sure mouth is clear and tongue is not blocking airway. Listen, look, feel for breath (3-4 sec.). If not breathing, or you are in doubt, start rescue breathing. If you suspect neck or back injury, pull open jaw without moving head (see inset).

2 Give two slow breaths.

Cover infant's nose and mouth with your mouth. Give two slow, *very gentle* breaths (puffs) of 1-1½ seconds each. Allow chest to rise and fall between breaths. NOTE: *Watch chest.* If chest does not rise and fall after 2 breaths, retilt head, pull chin up and try again. If airway is blocked, go to picture #3. If chest does rise and fall, *check pulse* as in picture #6.

3 Something in windpipe, use back blows.

Place baby face down over your forearm, resting arm on your thigh as shown, baby's head lower than chest. Support baby's head by holding jaw with your hand. Give 5 quick, firm back blows between the shoulders with the heel of your hand. If this does not work, go to #4.

4 Windpipe still blocked, use chest thrusts.

Turn baby over, still holding (supporting) head lower than chest. Place 2-3 fingers 1 finger width below nipple line and give 5 downward thrusts. Open baby's mouth by grasping tongue and lower jaw between thumb and fingers, and lifting. Only if you see object, gently sweep index finger (hooking motion) deeply into mouth at base of tongue to remove foreign body from throat.

NOTE: The use of latex gloves and mouth barrier with one-way valve (for rescue breathing) is recommended.

Not Breathing
No Pulse

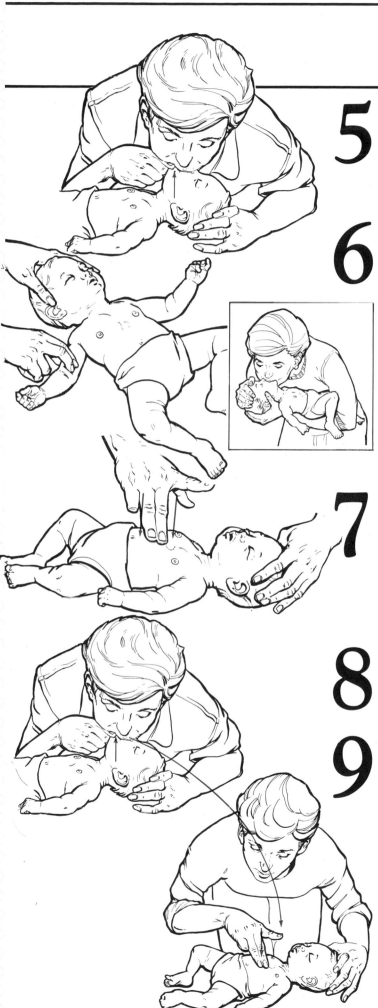

5 Repeat two slow breaths.

Tilt head back, lift chin, cover baby's nose and mouth with your mouth, and give two slow, *very gentle* breaths (puffs). Watch chest rise and fall. Repeat #3, #4 and #5 if necessary. Check for pulse.

6 Check for pulse on inside of the upper arm just above the bend in the elbow.

With the thumb on the outside of the arm, press middle and index fingers gently into the inside of the upper arm (see picture). Feel for pulse 3-4 seconds. *If no pulse,* start chest compressions (#7) along with rescue breathing. If baby has pulse, but is not breathing, continue one breath every 3 seconds for one minute (20 breaths/puffs). **Call 911/ambulance** (take baby with you while you call). Recheck breathing/pulse and continue one breath every 3 seconds until baby breathes on own or ambulance arrives.

7 Place 2-3 fingers on mid-breastbone 1 finger width below nipple line. Push down on chest ½"-1" (1.25 cm- 2.5 cm) - 5 times.

Push down on chest 5 times (rate of 100/min.). Let chest relax completely between downstrokes, without removing fingers from chest.

8 Give 1 slow breath.

Tilt head back. Lift chin. Cover baby's nose and mouth with your mouth. Give 1 slow, *very gentle* breath (puff). Make sure chest rises and falls.

9 Continue 5 chest compressions then 1 breath for 20 cycles. Call 911/ambulance.

Alternate 5 compressions and 1 breath for 20 cycles (1 minute). Call for ambulance (take baby with you or quickly return to baby). Recheck breathing/pulse (3-4 sec.). If there is a pulse but no breathing, give 1 breath/puff every 3 seconds. If no pulse, continue 5 chest compressions then 1 breath/puff. Continue until baby breathes on own or ambulance arrives. Recheck breathing/ pulse every few minutes. NOTE: Allow chest to rise and fall between breaths, let chest relax completely between downstrokes.

Choking

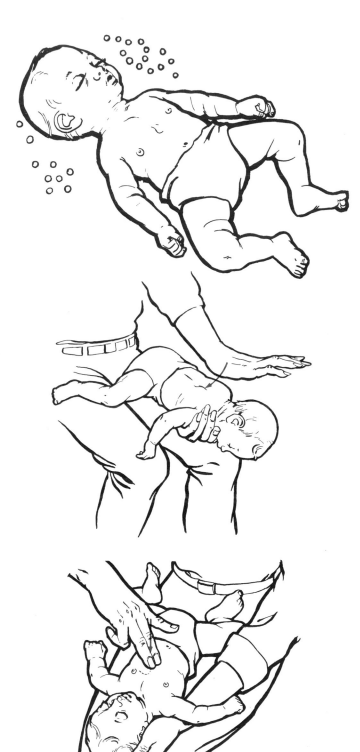

Do nothing if baby is coughing, breathing or "talking". Do not shake baby or hold upside down.

1 Recognize choking.

Use this procedure if you have seen or strongly suspect baby is choking on an object and if breathing is becoming more difficult. Lips may appear to be blue.

2 Something in windpipe, use back blows.

Place baby face down over your forearm, resting arm on your thigh as shown, baby's head lower than chest. Support baby's head by holding jaw with your hand. Give *5 quick, firm* back blows between the shoulders with the heel of your hand (if water or vomit comes up, clear mouth). If this does not work, go to #3.

3 Windpipe still blocked, use chest thrusts.

Turn baby over, still holding (supporting) head lower than chest. Place 2-3 fingers 1 finger width below nipple line and give 5 downward thrusts. Open baby's mouth by grasping tongue and lower jaw between thumb and fingers, and lifting. Only if you see object, gently sweep index finger (hooking motion) deeply into mouth at base of tongue to remove foreign body from throat. Repeat #2 and #3 until obstruction is gone or infant becomes unconscious.

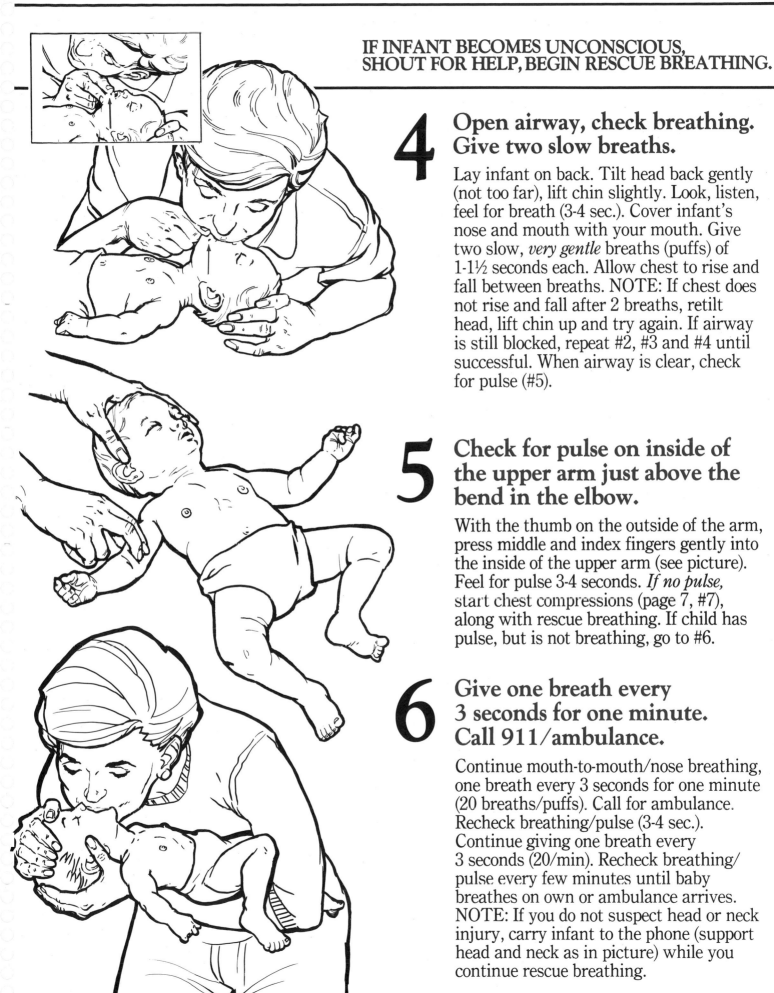

IF INFANT BECOMES UNCONSCIOUS,
SHOUT FOR HELP, BEGIN RESCUE BREATHING.

Choking

4 Open airway, check breathing. Give two slow breaths.

Lay infant on back. Tilt head back gently (not too far), lift chin slightly. Look, listen, feel for breath (3-4 sec.). Cover infant's nose and mouth with your mouth. Give two slow, *very gentle* breaths (puffs) of 1-1½ seconds each. Allow chest to rise and fall between breaths. NOTE: If chest does not rise and fall after 2 breaths, retilt head, lift chin up and try again. If airway is still blocked, repeat #2, #3 and #4 until successful. When airway is clear, check for pulse (#5).

5 Check for pulse on inside of the upper arm just above the bend in the elbow.

With the thumb on the outside of the arm, press middle and index fingers gently into the inside of the upper arm (see picture). Feel for pulse 3-4 seconds. *If no pulse,* start chest compressions (page 7, #7), along with rescue breathing. If child has pulse, but is not breathing, go to #6.

6 Give one breath every 3 seconds for one minute. Call 911/ambulance.

Continue mouth-to-mouth/nose breathing, one breath every 3 seconds for one minute (20 breaths/puffs). Call for ambulance. Recheck breathing/pulse (3-4 sec.). Continue giving one breath every 3 seconds (20/min). Recheck breathing/ pulse every few minutes until baby breathes on own or ambulance arrives. NOTE: If you do not suspect head or neck injury, carry infant to the phone (support head and neck as in picture) while you continue rescue breathing.

Seizure/Convulsion

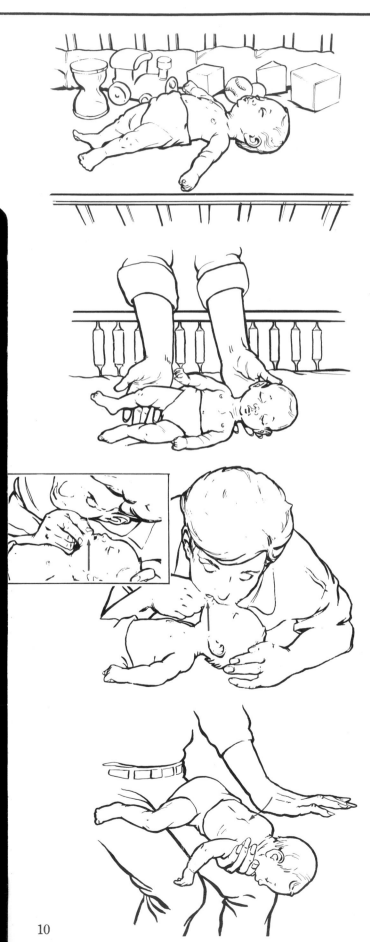

After seizure, make sure airway is clear and infant is breathing.

1 Infant is stiff.

Movements, if any, are jerky. Unconscious. Mouth may be frothy. Lips may appear to be blue.

2 Protect infant from injury.

Move harmful objects out of the way. Do not restrain baby or put anything in mouth. Protect the head.

3 Roll onto left side.

Protect airway if vomiting. SEIZURE MAY LAST 2-3 MINUTES.

AFTER SEIZURE, infant may be unconscious or confused. Make sure airway is open and baby is breathing. If not breathing, start rescue breathing (#4).

4 Open airway, check breathing. Give two slow breaths.

Lay infant on back. Tilt head back gently (not too far), lift chin slightly. Look, listen, feel for breath (3-4 sec.). If not breathing, cover infant's nose and mouth with your mouth. Give two slow, *very gentle* breaths (puffs) of 1-1½ seconds each. Allow chest to rise and fall between breaths. NOTE: If chest does not rise and fall after 2 breaths, retilt head, lift chin up and try again. If airway is blocked, go to picture #5. If chest does rise and fall, *check pulse* (#8).

5 Something in windpipe, use back blows.

Place baby face down over your forearm, resting arm on your thigh as shown, baby's head lower than chest. Support baby's head by holding jaw with your hand. Give 5 quick, firm back blows between the shoulders with the heel of your hand. If this does not work, go to #6.

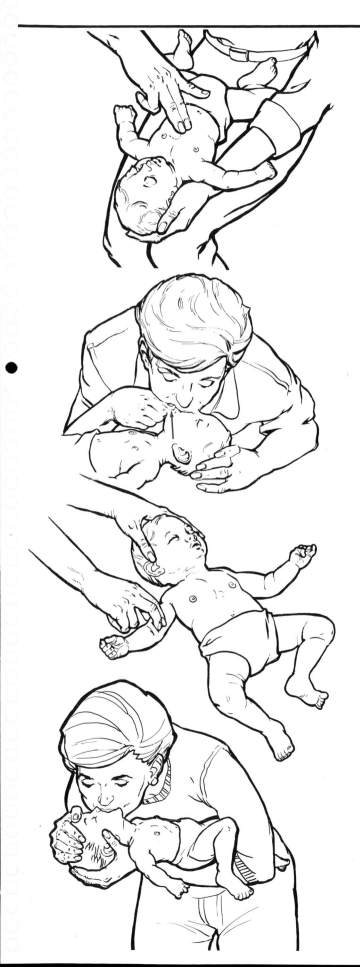

6 Windpipe still blocked, use chest thrusts.

Turn baby over, still holding (supporting) head lower than chest. Place 2-3 fingers 1 finger width below nipple line and give 5 downward thrusts. Open baby's mouth by grasping tongue and lower jaw between thumb and fingers, and lifting. Only if you see object, gently sweep index finger (hooking motion) deeply into mouth at base of tongue to remove foreign body from throat (never put fingers in mouth of seizing infant).

7 Repeat two slow breaths.

Tilt head back, lift chin, cover baby's nose and mouth with your mouth, and give two slow, *very gentle* breaths (puffs). Watch chest rise and fall. Repeat #5, #6 and #7 if necessary. Check for pulse.

8 Check for pulse on inside of the upper arm just above the bend in the elbow.

With the thumb on the outside of the arm, press middle and index fingers gently into the inside of the upper arm (see picture). Feel for pulse 3-4 seconds. *If no pulse,* start chest compressions (page 7, #7) along with rescue breathing. If child has pulse, but is not breathing, go to #9.

9 Give one breath every 3 seconds for one minute. Call 911/ambulance.

Continue mouth-to-mouth/nose breathing, one breath every 3 seconds for one minute (20 breaths/puffs). Call for ambulance. Recheck breathing/pulse (3-4 sec.). Continue giving one breath every 3 seconds (20/min). Recheck breathing/pulse every few minutes until baby breathes on own or ambulance arrives. NOTE: If you do not suspect head or neck injury, carry infant to the phone (support head and neck as in picture) while you continue rescue breathing.

Drowning

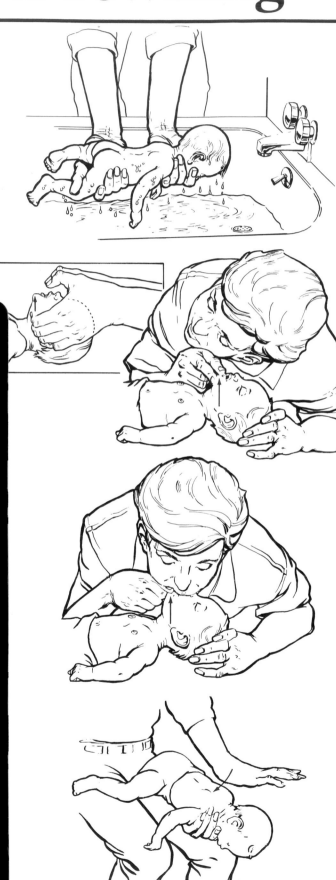

If infant is unconscious or does not respond, shout for help.

1 **Remove infant from water. Do nothing if coughing, breathing or "talking".**

2 **Open airway, check breathing.**
Lay infant on back. If you must roll infant on back, keep (support) head and neck in straight line. Tilt head back gently (not too far), lift chin slightly. Look, listen, feel for breath (3-4 sec.). If not breathing or you are in doubt, start rescue breathing (#3). If you suspect neck or back injury, pull open jaw without moving head (see inset).

3 **Give two slow breaths.**
Cover infant's nose and mouth with your mouth. Give two slow, *very gentle* breaths (puffs) of 1-1½ seconds each. Allow chest to rise and fall between breaths. NOTE: *Watch chest.* If chest does not rise and fall after 2 breaths, retilt head, lift chin up and try again. If airway is blocked, go to #4. If chest does rise and fall, *check pulse* as in #7.

4 **Something in windpipe, use back blows.**
Place baby face down over your forearm, resting arm on your thigh as shown, baby's head lower than chest. Support baby's head by holding jaw with your hand. Give 5 quick, firm back blows between the shoulders with the heel of your hand. If water or vomit comes up, clear mouth. If this does not work, go to #5.

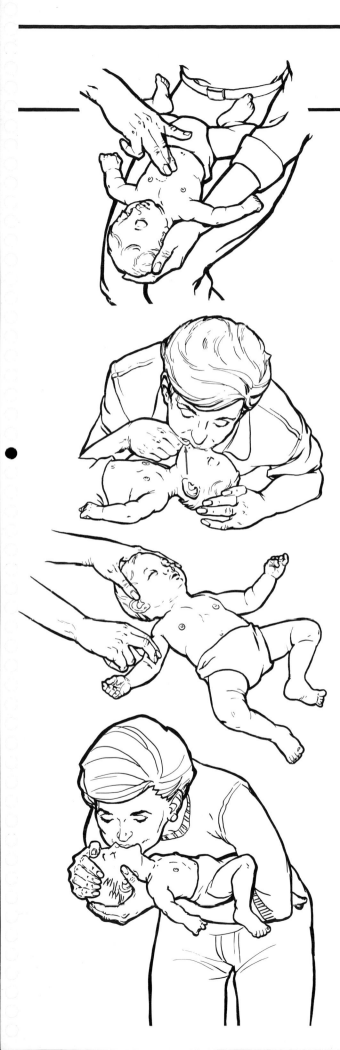

5 Windpipe still blocked, use chest thrusts.

Turn baby over, still holding (supporting) head lower than chest. Place 2-3 fingers 1 finger width below nipple line and give 5 downward thrusts. If water or vomit comes up, turn baby to side and clear mouth.

6 Repeat two slow breaths.

Tilt head back, lift chin, cover baby's nose and mouth with your mouth, and give two slow, *very gentle* breaths (puffs). Watch chest rise and fall. Repeat #4, #5 and #6 if necessary. Check for pulse.

7 Check for pulse on inside of the upper arm just above the bend in the elbow.

With the thumb on the outside of the arm, press middle and index fingers gently into the inside of the upper arm (see picture). Feel for pulse 3-4 seconds. *If no pulse,* start chest compressions (page 7, #7) along with rescue breathing. If child has pulse, but is not breathing, go to #8.

8 Give one breath every 3 seconds for one minute. Call 911/ambulance.

Continue mouth-to-mouth/nose breathing, one breath every 3 seconds for one minute (20 breaths/puffs). Call for ambulance. Recheck breathing/pulse (3-4 sec.). Continue giving one breath every 3 seconds (20/min). Recheck breathing/pulse every few minutes until baby breathes on own or ambulance arrives. NOTE: If you do not suspect head or neck injury, carry infant to the phone (support head and neck as in picture) while you continue rescue breathing.

Drowning

13

High Fever

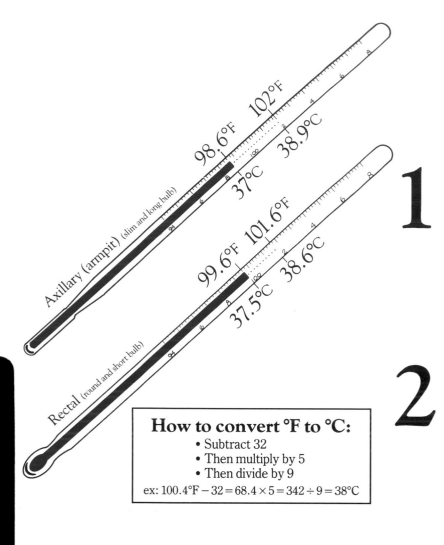

Any fever in an infant under 2 months is serious and should be seen by a doctor.

1 Recognize fever.

RECTAL TEMPERATURE is most reliable. Normal is 100.4°F (38°C). A high fever is 103.5°F (39.7°C).

AXILLARY (ARMPIT) TEMPERATURE is safest to take. Normal is 97°F to 98.6°F (36.1°C-37°C). A high fever is 101°F (38.3°C).

2 How to take an axillary (armpit) temperature.

Shake the thermometer, make sure it's not broken and that the top of the column is below 96°. Make sure that armpit is dry. Place bulb end of thermometer under arm and hold arm firmly against body for 4 minutes.

How to convert °F to °C:
- Subtract 32
- Then multiply by 5
- Then divide by 9

ex: $100.4°F - 32 = 68.4 \times 5 = 342 \div 9 = 38°C$

3 How to take a rectal temperature.

Shake the thermometer, make sure it's not broken and that the top of the column is below 96°. Lubricate the bulb of the thermometer with petroleum jelly. Spread the buttocks with the thumb and index finger of one hand so the anal opening is clearly seen. Insert just the bulb part of the thermometer into the center of the anal opening for 2 minutes. Keep the baby from moving so the thermometer doesn't break.

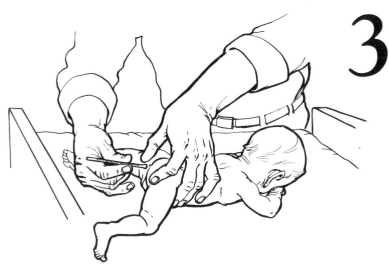

TREATMENT OF HIGH FEVERS

1. Take off any unnecessary clothing. Use light coverings if at all, so that body heat can escape, but do not let baby become chilled/avoid shivering.

2. Give baby plenty of cool things to drink.

3. Sponge baby with lukewarm water. Put baby in tub or sink of lukewarm, tepid water, not cold.

   DO NOT USE ICE, COLD WATER OR ALCOHOL SPONGING/BATHS

4. Give aspirin substitute (acetaminophen)** as instructed on label. If you have any questions, call your doctor or pharmacist.

5. Check temperature every ½ hour. Stop the sponging when the · temperature is down to 99.5° axillary or 102° rectally.

6. If you are worried or don't know what to do next, call your child's doctor for further advice.

   **WARNING: Aspirin used in conjunction with viral illnesses like colds, flu and chickenpox may increase the risk of Reyes Syndrome.

MENINGITIS AND OTHER SERIOUS/LIFE THREATENING INFECTIONS

Call your doctor or go the Emergency Room if any of these signs are present:

1. ALL INFANTS 2 MONTHS OR YOUNGER WITH FEVER MUST BE SEEN BY A DOCTOR.

2. Seizures/convulsions (see page 10).

3. Purple blotching or spotty rash.

4. Sleepy and hard to wake up (lethargic).

INFANT UNDER 3 MONTHS

Call your doctor or go to Emergency Room if any of these signs are present:

1. Lethargic, sleepy and hard to arouse.

2. Poor feeding.

3. Inconsolability (cries even when being held).

4. Increased irritability with handling/holding, does not want to be held.

5. Breathing rate more than 40/minute.

INFANT AGE 3-24 MONTHS

Call your doctor or go to Emergency Room if any of these signs are present:

1. Lethargic, sleepy and hard to arouse.

2. Poor feeding.

3. Inconsolability (cries even when being held).

4. Increased irritability with handling/holding, does not want to be held.

5. Breathing rate more than 40/minute.

AND

6. Less playful.

7. Less alert.

8. Less interactive with people/parents/environment.

High Fever

15

Bleeding

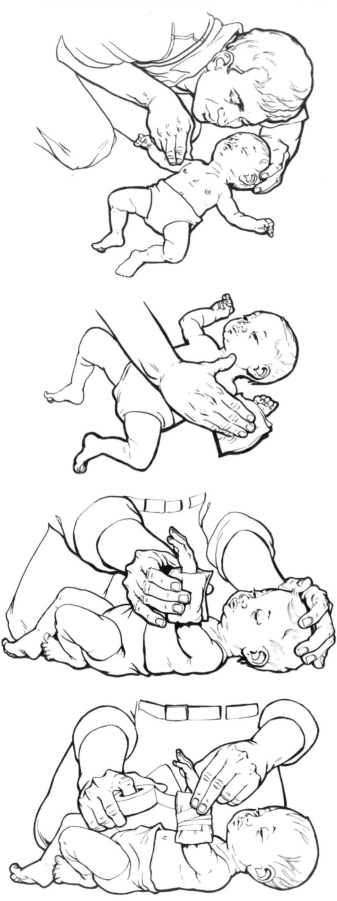

If infant is unconscious, does not respond, or bleeding appears to be serious, shout for help.

1 **Make sure baby is breathing and has a pulse BEFORE YOU STOP THE BLEEDING.**

Tilt head back gently (not too far), lift chin slightly. Listen, look, feel for breath (3-4 sec.) Check pulse (3-4 sec.) on inside of the upper arm just above the bend in the elbow. If not breathing or no pulse, turn immediately to page 6. If breathing and has pulse, go to #2.

2 **Apply direct pressure on bleeding wound with clean cloth.**

Do not remove dressing once it's on wound. If blood-soaked, place new dressing on old one.

3 **Keep pressure on.**

If wound is on arm or leg, apply pressure and elevate limb so that it is above the heart (unless limb is broken).

4 **Bandage firmly but not tightly** when bleeding is controlled.

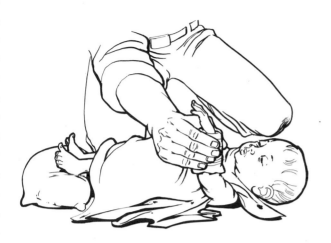

5 Care for shock.

If baby is cool, clammy or lethargic, elevate feet and keep warm. Note: Do not elevate feet if head injured, unconscious, chest injured, breathing difficulty. **Call 911/ambulance.**

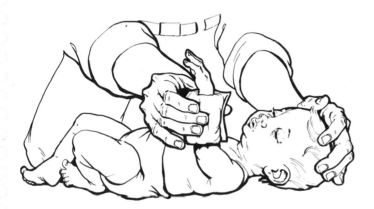

6 IF BLEEDING CONTINUES
Maintain firm pressure.

Press firmly as you continue direct pressure on wound. **Call 911/ambulance.**

A TOURNIQUET IS ALMOST NEVER NEEDED AND IS DANGEROUS. Even bleeding arteries can almost always be controlled with pressure.

Bleeding

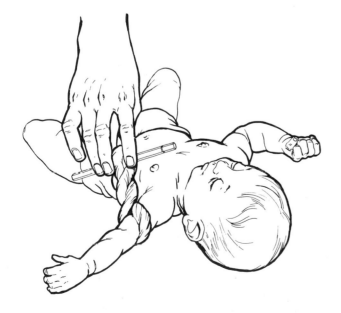

7 Use a tourniquet ONLY AS THE LAST RESORT. Appropriate only when all other methods do not stop the bleeding.

Wrap a piece of cloth above wound, between wound and heart. Twist a stick around ties just tight enough to stop flow of blood to wound. Hold or tie cloth.

NOTE THE TIME. NEVER LOOSEN TOURNIQUET. CALL AMBULANCE/ TRANSPORT TO HOSPITAL.

Vomiting/Diarrhea (DEHYDRATION)

1 **Look for signs of dehydration (loss of body fluids).**

1. Diminished urination (less frequent, fewer/less soaked diapers)
2. Sunken eyes
3. Sunken soft spot in infant's skull
4. Drowsy, lethargic
5. Rapid or slower breathing
6. Diminished or no tears
7. Dryness in mouth
8. Less skin firmness
9. Weight loss (the loss of as little as 5% of infant's weight is a sign of serious dehydration)

2 **Give clear liquids frequently and in small amounts.**

Water, flat carbonated beverages, flavored gelatin water, commercial electrolyte solutions (available from your pharamacist).

3 **Dehydration in infants is serious.**

It can happen as quickly as 12 hours after the start of vomiting, diarrhea, or prolonged high fever. If unable to get baby to keep liquids in, call your doctor or take baby to the Emergency Room.

VOMITING

Do not give antivomiting medicines to infant.

1. Prolonged or severe vomiting can cause dehydration in as little as 12 hours, and can be life threatening.

2. If there is very forceful (projectile) vomiting in the first 3 months, the baby must be seen by a doctor.

3. Do not give baby any milk products or solid foods.

4. Give clear liquids frequently, in small amounts.
   Tablespoonfuls of liquid, for example. Liquids include water, flat carbonated beverages, flavored gelatin water, commercial electrolyte solutions (available from your pharmacist). Do not allow infant to take large amounts, or will just vomit again.

5. Call doctor or go to Emergency Room if infant's frequent vomiting lasts more than 12 hours, there are of signs of dehydration (see facing page), or vomiting makes child unable to take needed/prescribed medication.

DIARRHEA

Do not give antidiarrhea medicines to infant.

1. Watch for signs of dehydration (see facing page).
   Dehydration can occur in as little as 12 hours and can be life threatening.

2. Frequency and amount of diarrhea reflect the severity of the problem. Small amounts of diarrhea are common in infants. If you have a question, call your doctor.

3. Do not give any milk products or solid foods.

4. Stop any new or recently started foods (they may be the cause).

5. Do not stop needed/prescribed medications without your doctor's permission.

6. Give clear liquids frequently, in small amounts.
   Tablespoonfuls of liquid, for example. Liquids include water, flat carbonated beverages, flavored gelatin water, commercial electrolyte solutions (available from your pharmacist).

7. Call doctor or take to Emergency Room if there are signs of dehydration (see facing page), *frequent* diarrhea that lasts more than 12 hours, or there is blood in bowel movement.

Vomiting & Diarrhea

19

Burns

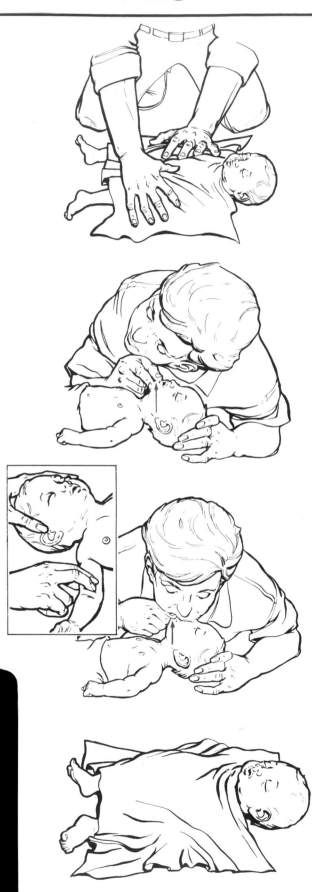

Shout for help!

HEAT BURNS — FIRE OR HOT LIQUIDS

1 Stop the burning.

Roll infant on ground until flames are out (Stop, Drop & Roll), or use water.

2 Make sure baby is responsive and is breathing.

Tilt head back gently (not too far), lift chin slightly. Look, listen, feel for breath (3-4 sec.). If not breathing, start rescue breathing (#3).

3 Give two slow breaths. Check for pulse.

Cover infant's nose and mouth with your mouth. Give two slow, *very gentle* breaths into baby's mouth. Check for pulse (3-4 sec.) on inside of the upper arm just above the bend in the elbow. If no pulse, turn to page 7, #7. If pulse but not breathing, give one breath every 3 seconds for one minute. **Call 911/ambulance** (carry infant with you). Recheck breathing/pulse, continue giving one breath every 3 seconds until baby breathes on own or ambulance arrives. Recheck breathing/pulse every few minutes.

4 Cover with clean, dry sheet.

Do not use ointment, salves or any other medication. Do not remove blisters, skin. Remove hot/burned clothes that come off easily. Do not remove clothing stuck to skin. For all blistered, charred or scorched burns; for burns to the crotch, hands, feet or joints; for smoke inhalation by baby - see a doctor.
CALL 911/AMBULANCE

SEE PAGE 24 FOR LESS SEVERE BURNS

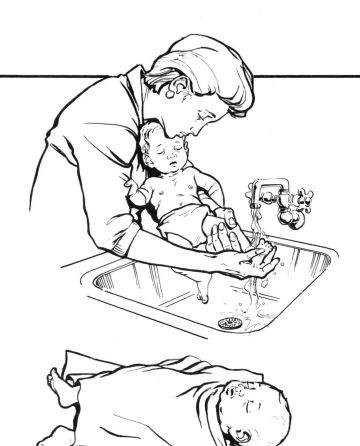

CHEMICAL BURNS

1 **Rinse/brush chemicals off skin, eyes, FAST.**

Seconds count. Get baby's clothes off and use shower/hose off/buckets of water immediately. Rinse for no less than 30 minutes.

2 **Make sure baby is breathing and has pulse.**

See pictures #2 and #3 on opposite page and follow instructions.

3 **Cover with clean, dry sheet.**

Do not use ointments, salves or any other medication. Do not remove blisters, skin.

CALL 911/AMBULANCE

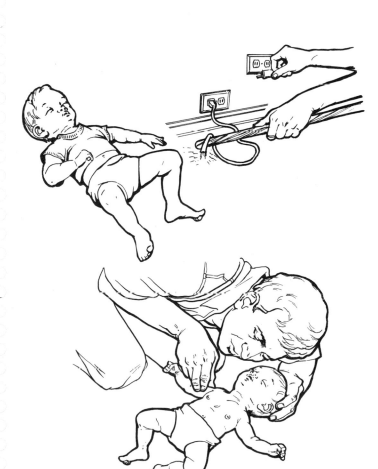

ELECTRICAL BURNS/INJURY

1 **Do not touch baby until electricity is turned off. Remove baby from source of electricity.**

Unplug cord, turn off electric current.

2 **Make sure baby is breathing and has pulse.**

See pictures #2 and #3 on opposite page and follow instructions. Note: Cover and keep warm.

CALL 911/AMBULANCE

Burns

21

Head, Neck and Back Injury

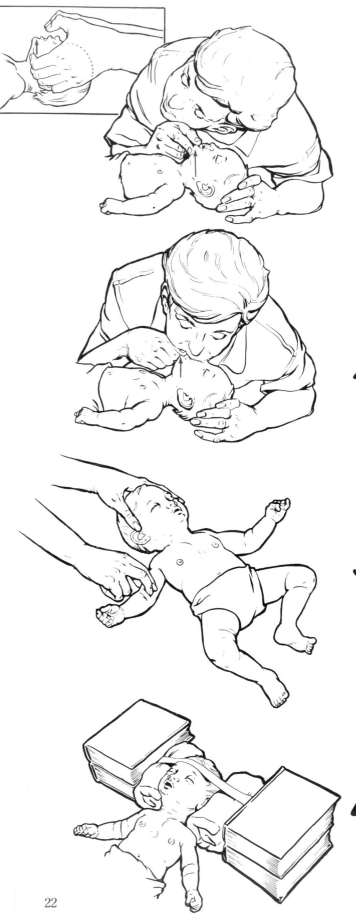

Very gently tap or shake infant. If infant does not respond, shout for help.

1 **Assume neck/spinal injury. DO NOT MOVE OR ELEVATE HEAD OR MOVE INFANT UNLESS IN LIFE-THREATENING DANGER. Make sure infant is breathing.**

Open airway by pulling jaw forward *without moving head or neck* (see inset). Look, listen, feel for breath (3-4 sec.). If not breathing or you are in doubt, start rescue breathing (#2).

2 **Give two slow breaths.**

Cover infant's nose and mouth with your mouth. Give two slow, *very gentle* breaths (puffs) of 1-1½ seconds each. Allow chest to rise and fall between breaths. NOTE: *Watch chest.* If chest does not rise and fall after 2 breaths, retilt head, lift chin up and try again. If airway is blocked, go to page 6, #3. If chest does rise and fall, *check pulse.*

3 **Check for pulse on inside of the upper arm just above the bend in the elbow.**

Check for pulse (3-4 sec.) on inside of the upper arm just above the bend in the elbow. If no pulse, turn to page 7, #7. If pulse but not breathing, give one breath every 3 seconds for one minute. **Call 911/ambulance,** quickly return to baby. Recheck breathing/pulse, continue giving one breath every 3 seconds until baby breathes on own or ambulance arrives. Recheck breathing/pulse every few minutes.

4 **DO NOT MOVE OR ELEVATE HEAD.**

Make it so baby's head cannot move. Place rolled up towels on either side of head. Anchor towels with heavy object or sand bags as pictured. Tape forehead down to floor if possible, keep from moving.

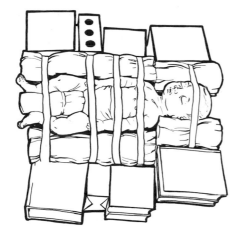

5 Keep entire body from moving.

Place rolled up towels around rest of body and anchor with heavy objects or sand bags as pictured.

DO NOT MOVE INFANT UNLESS YOU ABSOLUTELY HAVE TO.

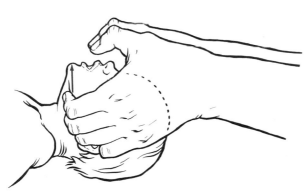

6 Make sure infant is breathing.

If infant is having difficulty breathing (loud/snoring breathing) or is unconscious, open airway by pulling jaw forward without moving head or neck. Look, listen, feel for breath (3-4 sec.). If not breathing or you are in doubt, start rescue breathing (#2 & #3). If infant is breathing, help keep airway open if necessary.

THINGS TO DO AND WATCH FOR AFTER A HEAD INJURY

1. No pain medication other than aspirin substitute (acetaminophen) should be taken.
2. Apply ice pack over swollen or painful areas (if it doesn't make baby scream or cry).
3. Child should rest.
4. Awaken child every 4 hours to check for signs listed below.

CONTACT YOUR CHILD'S DOCTOR OR TRANSPORT TO EMERGENCY ROOM IMMEDIATELY IF ANY OF THE FOLLOWING OCCUR:

1. If child is unusually sleepy and/or harder to waken than usual.
2. If nausea or vomiting, which is common right away, persists.
3. If child has unequal pupils.
4. If child has more difficulty keeping balance than usual.
5. If child seems confused or displays unusual behavior.
6. If blood is coming from ear.
7. If watery fluid is coming from ear or nose.
8. If child has slow pulse (less than 60/minute) or abnormal breathing.

Head, Neck & Back Injuries

23

Other Serious Illness

HEAT BURNS

1. First-degree burns (redness like sunburn, pain). Apply cold (water, ice pack). Do not use ointments or butter.

2. Second-degree burns (blisters, raw areas develop). Immerse in cold water, then dry and cover with sterile gauze or cloth. Treat for shock (page 17, #5) and seek medical attention. Do not break blisters or apply ointments or butter.

3. Third-degree burns (leathery, charring and often little pain). See page 20, #2 - #4.

DIFFICULTY BREATHING

1. Child may appear blue and has a lot of trouble breathing (noisy, rapid).

2. May have barking cough.

3. May have fever.

4. May tend to be quiet.

5. May not want to lie down flat.

6. May be drooling.

7. Any of these symptoms may be serious. Call baby's doctor or go to Emergency Room immediately.

FEBRILE SEIZURES

Most seizures in young children are related to fever –the result of a sudden rise/change in temperature. While frightening, most turn out to be not serious. ALL first seizures must be seen by a doctor, to make sure it is not something more serious, like meningitis. Even if your child has had febrile seizures in the past, you should call your doctor if one occurs.

BARKING COUGH AND NOISY BREATHING (CROUP & BRONCHIOLITIS)

1. If difficulty breathing, always call doctor or go to Emergency Room.

2. *Croup,* with barking cough (like a seal): Place child in a room with high moisture – steamy bathroom, room with vaporizer.

3. Try to keep child quiet – crying will increase coughing.

4. Bronchiolitis usually begins as a cold with cough and runny nose. Over several days difficulty breathing develops.

5. Wheezing may progress to grunting in order to breathe.

6. Flaring out of nostrils and chest/abdomen being sucked in with breathing are seen.

7. Bronchiolitis is serious, and infants with these signs must be seen by their doctor or in the Emergency Room.

NOSEBLEED

1. Pinch nostrils just below bony bridge of nose. Hold tight pressure for at least 5-10 minutes.

2. If you cannot control the nosebleed, go to Emergency Room or call ambulance immediately.

BROKEN BONES

1. STABILIZE BROKEN LIMB

Splint it as it lies. Materials you can use as splints include rolled up newspaper, magazine, wood, pillow, rolled up towel.

2. BROKEN COLLAR BONE, SHOULDER, ELBOW

Place arm in sling to support arm. Bind to body. Place icebag over break, NOT directly on skin.

3. BROKEN ARM, WRIST

Splint arm or wrist with rolled up newspaper, magazine, or wood. Tie securely, place in sling as above. Bind to body. Place icebag over break, NOT directly on skin.

4. BROKEN LEG

Splint leg with rolled up newspaper, magazine, or wood. Use pillow or cloth for padding. Tie securely. Place icebag over break, NOT directly on skin.

5. BROKEN ANKLE OR FOOT

Splint ankle or foot with a pillow. Tie securely. Place icebag over break, NOT directly on skin.

COLIC

1. Daily periods of crying and irritability that may last for hours, have no obvious cause, usually in late afternoon or evening.

2. Usually begins in second to third week of life, and usually goes on for about three months.

3. Crying that may become piercing screams as if the baby is in pain. Baby may draw up its legs and clench its fists, abdomen may look distended, and baby may pass gas.

TREATMENT FOR COLIC

1. Look for possible signs of other illness or cause for discomfort — open diaper pin, sores, bad diaper rash.

2. Offer a feeding to see if baby is simply hungry. Make sure bottle's nipple is full, to keep child from swallowing too much air.

3. Temporary, brief relief can often come from cuddling, rhymthmic motions such as rocking/carrying/riding in the car.

4. You can try applying GENTLE heat to the abdomen.

5. NO definite cure is available, but the symptoms almost always disappear about 3 months after they start.

6. Call your doctor if you are unsure/have any questions.

Other Serious Illness

25

ABOUT THE AUTHORS

Stephen N. Vogel, M.D.

Dr. Vogel was one of the first physicians in the United States specially trained in the field of Emergency Medicine. He is a member of the Departments of Medicine and Department of Surgery at Northwestern University. Since 1975 he has been an attending physician in the Department of Emergency Medicine, Evanston Hospital, Evanston, Illinois.

David H. Manhoff

Mr. Manhoff was trained in the late 1960's as a Combat Medical Corpsman in the United States Army. For the past 24 years, Mr. Manhoff has been an advertising writer. He is currently an Executive Creative Director of an advertising agency in Chicago, Illinois. He, his wife and two children, one of whom was the inspiration for this book, live in Wilmette, Illinois.